Vegetarian

Discover Delicious Vegetarian Recipes Along With Secrets To Becoming Super Healthy With A Nutritious Vegetarian Diet

By Ace McCloud
Copyright © 2014

Disclaimer

The information provided in this book is designed to provide helpful information on the subjects discussed. This book is not meant to be used, nor should it be used, to diagnose or treat any medical condition. For diagnosis or treatment of any medical problem, consult your own physician. The publisher and author are not responsible for any specific health or allergy needs that may require medical supervision and are not liable for any damages or negative consequences from any treatment, action, application or preparation, to any person reading or following the information in this book. Any references included are provided for informational purposes only. Readers should be aware that any websites or links listed in this book may change.

Table of Contents

Introduction 6
Chapter 1: What Exactly is a Vegetarian? 7
Chapter 2: Why So Many People Choose Vegetarianism 8
Chapter 3: The Vegetarian Food Pyramid and a Few Food Recommendations 11
Chapter 4: Tasty Vegetarian Recipes for Appetizers and Snacks 15
Chapter 5: Tasty Vegetarian Recipes for Lunch and Dinner 20
Chapter 6: Delicious and Healthy Smoothies 26
Chapter 7: Fitness Tips for Vegetarians 29
Conclusion 31
My Other Books and Audio Books 32

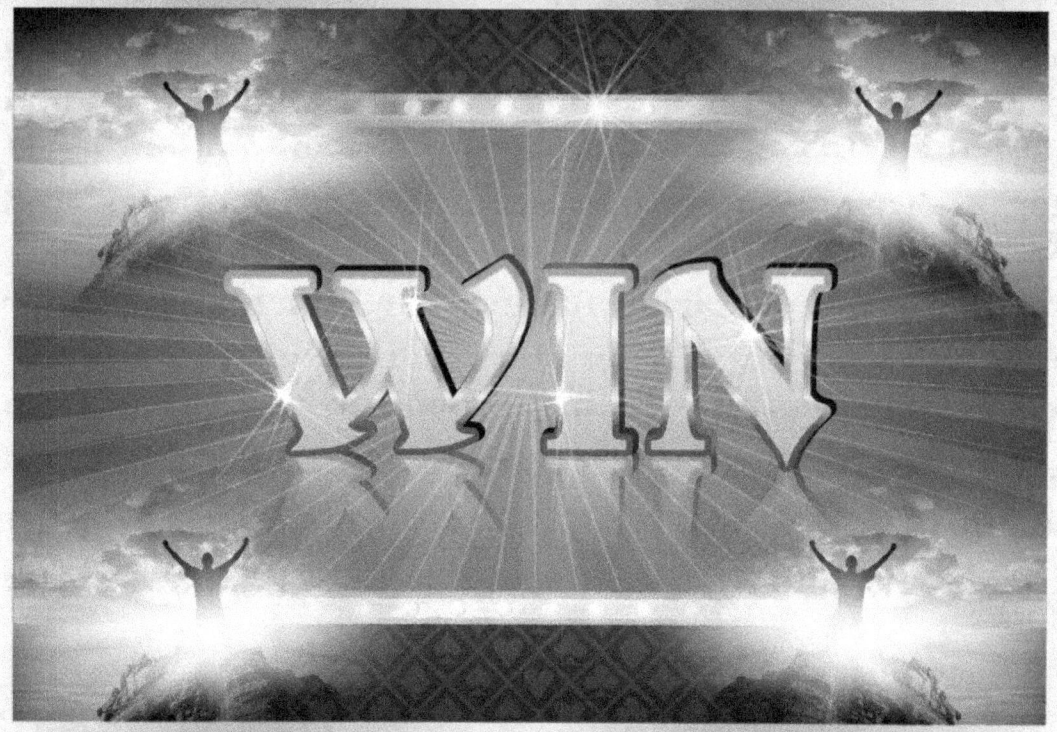

Be sure to check out my website for all my Books and Audio books.

www.AcesEbooks.com

Introduction

I want to thank you and congratulate you for buying the book, "Vegetarian Diet Recipes And Cooking – Learn How To Be Healthy And Fit With A Nutritious Vegetarian Lifestyle That Promotes Health, Good Living, Great Food, And Fitness"

This book contains proven steps and strategies on how to maximize the benefits of vegetarianism. Some of the things you will discover in this book include the best and healthiest foods to eat, delicious recipes, incredible smoothie recipes, healthy living tips, and lots of delicious vegetarian recipes with easy preparation instructions!

If you are truly looking for more energy, better health, or to just have a more healthy and enjoyable life, this is the book for you!

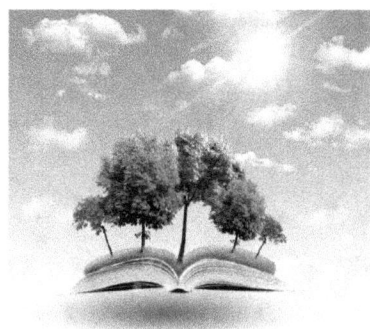

Chapter 1: What Exactly is a Vegetarian?

From various types of experts to vegetarians themselves, people often have different definitions of vegetarianism. However, a consensus can often be met. For the purposes of this book, a vegetarian is defined as someone who does not eat meat, but is lacto-ovo, meaning a vegetarian who consumes eggs and dairy, the products of animals, but not the animal itself. A vegan, on the other hand, tries to never consume any type of meat and often refuses to wear animal products such as fur and leather. Vegans also try not to consume any animal-made products such as honey, dairy, or eggs. Being a vegetarian is certainly a lifestyle choice, not simply a diet, but it doesn't need to be difficult, especially when one considers the great benefits of being a vegetarian.

Many people are worried that if they don't eat meat that they won't have energy or the protein necessary to work out and build muscle. With all of the careful studies that have been done and the variety of all natural protein sources available, worry no more. Vegetarian diets have been shown over and over again in study after study to be healthy and in many ways healthier than diets with meat in them. You can build and maintain great muscle strength as a vegetarian and greatly increase your energy levels. There are even vegetarians and vegans who blog and write books about their major health and fitness successes.

The health benefits of vegetarianism are numerous. Some of the more notable benefits of being a vegetarian include: a lower risk of becoming obese, a decreased chance of lung cancer, reduced hypertension, reduced chances of getting gallstones, a reduction in the chances of becoming an alcoholic, reduced chances of coronary heart disease, and much more! In fact, just being a vegetarian can decrease your overall chances of getting various diseases, protect you against various types of cancer and increase your chances of living longer!

Chapter 2: Why So Many People Choose Vegetarianism

If you're reading this book, you may be considering becoming a vegetarian, have already decided to make the change, or you're already a vegetarian who would like to learn more. This book offers information for you that is relevant and helpful no matter what stage you are in.

For those considering becoming vegetarian, there are a myriad of reasons for making the shift. One reason is to lose weight, and people who are vegetarian tend to be thinner than non-vegetarians. One theory for this statistic is that vegetarians restrict what they eat, but not how much they eat. Therefore, if you choose healthy meals and can eat until you're full; it is less likely that you will splurge later on because you are not hungry. However, just switching to a vegetarian diet won't make you lose weight. You need to make sure you are sticking to healthy choices that are lower in fat and not overindulging in sweets. Simply following a lifestyle everyday can help in paying attention to what you are eating and lead to better food selection choices. Along with weight loss there are the many nutritional benefits of a vegetarian diet that have been shown over and over again, which I'll go into more detail in Chapter 3.

Another reason many people switch diets is for environmental reasons. Farming animals for consumption emits a large amount of greenhouse gases, uses a lot more water and land, not to mention the overfishing of the oceans, compared to growing vegetables and grains. "In 2006, the UN calculated that the combined climate change emissions of animals bred for their meat were about 18% of the global total – more than cars, planes and all other forms of transport put together."

Another reason some people convert to vegetarianism is to advocate for the humane treatment of animals. It is not a secret that many factory farmed animals are put in squalid living conditions before being killed. For this reason some people only eat local farm meat instead of becoming vegetarian, but many people don't believe it's necessary to kill animals in and simply abstain from eating them.

Vegetarianism can also save money by cutting out the cost of meat. Relatedly, you can start eating more in season. Eating in season, eating what produce is locally available, is much less expensive than buying foods that are shipped from a long distance.

What are some steps you can take to ensure an easy interaction with non-vegetarians in food situations? One major courtesy when eating outside of your home is to plan ahead by letting your host know you're a vegetarian. Some people may have bad associations with vegetarians or not understand the diet.

You could also prepare the meal yourself in many situations and eat healthy while saving money at the same time.

If you travel a lot or eat out a lot, it's easy to slip into eating "junk" food. Again, planning ahead is a great solution. If your problem is that you eat out all week, while not making healthy choices, plan ahead. Over the weekend make a meal plan for the week (for example, I'm having lentil shepherd's pie with a side of broccoli on Monday, I'm having quinoa stuffed squash on Tuesday, etc.) The meal plan doesn't even need to be this rigid, you can pick out a number of appetizing meals and decide what you cook depending on how you feel each night. After making your meal choices for the week, head to the grocery store for everything that won't spoil by the end of the week. As the week progresses you simply need to pick up a few fresh items at a time. Another great option is to make your meals in bulk batches ahead of time. Simply refrigerate or freeze the extra servings, allowing for quick preparation time in the future.

When converting to more of a plant based diet one thing to consider is vitamins and minerals, which I'll hopefully make easy for you. It is incredibly important to know what foods you can naturally get these essential vitamins and minerals from. While most people can get the majority of their nutrition from the food they eat, it is important to pay attention to the following vitamins and minerals as a vegetarian because they are especially important. Check with your doctor if you think you may be deficient in a particular vitamin.

Vitamins, Minerals and Other Dietary Considerations that Vegetarians should be aware of:

Vitamin B12-produces red blood cells and prevents anemia. This can be very hard to find in the vegetarian diet. Again, most of the vitamins and minerals we need are easily found in the diet, but this is one where you probably want to find a supplement. My favorite form is B-12 that I personally take is: Jarrows B-12.

Calcium is another mineral to keep an eye on, as it contributes to strong teeth and bones. This can be obtained from dairy and dark greens such as spinach or kale. In supplement form here is a good choice: Nature Made Calcium Supplement.

Vitamin D-aids bone health. Many dairy as well as other products are fortified with vitamin D. You also naturally absorb this vitamin from the sun. In supplement form a good choice is: Vitafusion Chewable Calcium with Vitamin D

Iron-composes red blood cells. This can be obtained from dried beans, whole grains, and dark leafy greens. A good trick to know is to eat iron-rich foods with vitamin C as it is better absorbed. In supplement form here is a good choice: Nature Made Iron Supplement

Omega 3 fatty acids-contributes to heart health. This can be obtained from eggs, walnuts and ground flaxseed. However, this is one of the rare instances where the fatty acid is often hard to get naturally from a vegetarian diet. In this case it's a good idea to consider an omega 3 or omega complex (3,6,9) supplement. Kirkland Omega 3 Natural Fish Oil is a good choice.

Protein-contributes to healthy skin, bones, muscles, and organs. This can be obtained from eggs, dairy, plant sources, lentils, nuts and seeds. My favorite protein drink that works great is: **Muscle Milk**.

Zinc-contributes to cell division and the formation of proteins. Vegetarians can find zinc in cheeses and soy. Also, here is a good supplement with Zinc in it: Nature Made Calcium Magnesium Zinc.

To be clear and hopeful for vegetarians, for the most part, if you educate yourself (such as reading this book, congratulations!) and cook/eat healthy, balanced meals, take the occasional supplement, then you probably will not have a problem getting the far majority of the vitamins and minerals you need, but it can never hurt to ensure abundance with supplements.

Chapter 3: The Vegetarian Food Pyramid and a Few Food Recommendations

All fruits, vegetables, beans and grains are considered vegetarian. However, some are better for your general health and some are even better for your health as a vegetarian. For example, dark leafy greens which contain iron and antioxidants are always a great choice.

The distinct difference in a vegetarian's diet versus an omnivore's diet is that lacto-ovo vegetarians don't consume animals in any form (for example, broth):
-Beef
-Chicken
-Pig
-Turkey
-Duck
-Any type of seafood such as fish, crabs, lobster or shrimp
-Or any type of wild caught game, etc.

In general, as an article in the American Journal of Nutrition about the vegetarian food pyramid recommends, whole wheat, whole grains and soy can be used as a possible alternative to meat. These foods are fortified with vitamin D, calcium and B12. Dark leafy greens, yellow and green vegetables, both cooked and raw, are excellent choices as well. Nuts and seeds are recommended, but try to stay away from deep fried nuts. The best oils are high in monounsaturated fats and hydrogenated fats should be avoided. What are some recommended vegetarian protein sources on the pyramid? Six Pack Shortcuts' YouTube video 7 Best Protein Sources For Vegetarians suggests some great protein sources.

The following is a list of what are often called "superfoods," named so because they have so many healthy properties. These foods may give you ideas for what to incorporate into your cooking or to utilize just as a snack. Here is a quick note on fiber, which is a great benefit of vegetables. A major US study followed 10,000 adults, with 19 years of follow up and tracked fiber intake the whole time. The study clearly revealed that those people who ate the most fiber had a scientifically significant lower risk of heart disease and stroke than those who ate little fiber.

Almonds
Almonds contain monounsaturated fats, which is considered a healthy fat, especially for vegetarians, and recommended by nutritionists when consumed in moderation. Almonds also contain magnesium, which lowers blood pressure and possibly reducing kidney disease, potassium, and anti-ageing properties. Here are some great almonds you can find online: Blue Diamond Almonds.

Apples
Apples have many nutritional benefits (though they are high in sugar). This is considered a superfood, partially because of the pectin in it that is a natural fiber

and that alleviates indigestion, gout, rheumatism, arthritis, and lowers cholesterol and reduces hangovers. Apples are also a great food to be used to help with diarrhea. There are many others benefits to apples as well and a highly recommended food source in any diet.

Avocado
Although people are sometimes wary of avocados because of their high fat content, most of the fat is monounsaturated, the good kind we talked about earlier. Avocados are a good source of vitamin E, which helps keep the heart healthy. Just 1 avocado aids with a healthy nervous system. Additionally, women taking the pill or anyone taking antibiotics, reap the benefits of vitamin B6, which is linked to depression.

Beans
Beans really pack a punch. In addition to their well-known benefits from fiber, beans have been linked to lowering cholesterol. Furthermore, they are a great preventative, as studies show they protect against osteoporosis, heart disease, diabetes and several cancers.

Blueberries & Berries
Blueberries are beloved by experts as they've been shown to effectively protect the body from premature ageing, heart disease, cancer, high cholesterol and degenerative diseases. Luckily all berries protect against cancer, but in addition to blueberries, blackberries, are a major gem because they have been shown to slow down the growth rate of certain cancers.

Watermelon
Watermelons boost a huge dose of antioxidants in addition to vitamins A and C. Watermelon also contains lycopene, the cancer fighting agent found in a number of fruits.

Yellow and Orange Vegetables such as sweet potatoes, carrots, bell peppers, squash, and pumpkin generally help benefit vision, skin, bones, heart and immune function.

Red Vegetables such as red onions, beets, radishes, red peppers, tomatoes, and rhubarb have been shown to boost immunity and benefit the memory.

The **purple colored vegetables** such as purple onions, purple cabbage, and eggplant have been shown to have anti-inflammatory properties.

Green vegetables such as spinach, kale, broccoli, asparagus, collard greens, brussel sprouts, swiss chard, celery, and peas, can help with macular degeneration.

Broccoli

I don't think broccoli is given the due it deserves. It contains fiber, calcium, vitamins A, K and D along with antioxidants. It also has a powerful detoxification effect as well as fighting many diseases such as cancer, cataracts, heart disease, arthritis and ulcers.

Carrots
Carrots are an excellent source of beta carotene, which is converted into vitamin A. Vitamin A is an extremely important part of the function of skin.

Chickpeas
Chickpeas perform a double duty as a vegetable. They not only pack in fiber, vitamins and minerals such as potassium, but they are a good source of protein for vegetarians. Chickpeas lower cholesterol, lower blood pressure and can help prevent heart disease, stroke, as well as diabetes.

Garlic
Garlic truly is a healing plant. It has been shown to have antiviral, anti-fungal and antibiotic abilities. Additionally, it may protect against heart disease and blood clots while helping to lower blood pressure and it can even act as an anti-carcinogen.

Kiwi fruit
Surprisingly, to some, kiwis have a huge amount of vitamin C and potassium in them. However, what is considered the best part of this fruit is its lutein content, an antioxidant that protects against macular degeneration. If you are at all worried about your eyesight or would like to know all the best strategies for keeping your eyesight in peak condition, be sure to check out my book: **Eyesight and Vision Cure**.

Leafy greens
Leafy greens contain all sorts contain vitamin C, beta-carotene, folic acid, calcium and fiber. However, the best superfoods of the leafy greens tend to be the dark leafy greens. In particular, spinach, kale, collards and broccoli are rich in antioxidants. As talked about with the kiwi fruit, research has also shown that a high intake of dark leafy greens reduces the risk of cataracts and macular degeneration while as an added bonus of being an anti-carcinogen as well. Dark leafy greens have also been found to be good as a preventative measure for osteoporosis. If you would like to know more about osteoporosis, be sure to check out my book: **Osteoporosis Cure**.

Oranges
Oranges are known for being high in vitamin C and beta-carotene. They also are good disease-fighters; including helping prevent heart disease, stroke and various types of cancer such as mouth, throat and stomach cancers.

Sweet potato

Sweet potatoes are stacked with vitamin E as well as vitamin A, C, B6, iron, and potassium. These vitamins provide a range of benefits such as skin health linked to vitamin A or a boost to your immune system that is provided by vitamin C.

Tomatoes

Tomatoes are your best bet for lycopene, which in studies has been shown to be an anti-carcinogen, especially for breast and prostate cancer. But the benefits don't stop there. In studies completed with older patients, lycopene has been shown to protect against vision loss and heart disease as well.

Nuts

Most nuts contain many brain and heart healthy substances. They are composed of unsaturated fats, which, as discussed before, lower cholesterol. Nuts also contain fiber, which is beneficial in digestion, and vitamin E, which helps prevent heart attacks. The omega-3 fatty acids in nuts have also been shown to be beneficial in lowering the chance of acquiring Alzheimer's disease. If you want o ensure that you are getting all the great omega-3 fatty acids you need, here is a great product: Nature Made Omega 3 supplement.

Chapter 4: Tasty Vegetarian Recipes for Appetizers and Snacks

Now the tasty and healthy recipes! One major thing that I've always heard that helps new vegetarians is substituting vegetables in recipes for meat slowly. For example, if you like shepherd's pie, try replacing the ground beef with lentils.

If you're trying to lose weight, being a vegetarian is a great way to do this. Vegetables take up a lot of volume but they don't have the fat and calories that other foods, in particular meat, do. So pile your plate up with vegetables, feel full, and reap the benefits of a vegetarian diet.

First a link to a YouTube video about making protein bars from scratch by NATURALGC: Healthiest Homemade Protein Bar.

Avocado hummus
- 1 can of chickpeas, drained and rinsed
- 1 avocado, cut into smaller pieces
- 1 clove of garlic, cut into smaller pieces
- 1 Tbsp. olive oil, plus more if needed for consistency and to drizzle on top
- 1/2 tsp. salt
- 1/4 tsp. cayenne pepper, plus more to drizzle on top

1. Juice ½-1 lime, to your taste, and add to a food processor. Add the rest of the ingredients to the food processor
2. Process all of the ingredients until desired consistency is reached. Drizzle with olive oil and add a dash of cayenne pepper.

Stuffed Avocado:
- 2 ripe avocados (or more if you have extra stuffing left)
- 1/2 Cup dry quinoa
- 1 can black beans, rinsed and drained
- 1/2 red onion, chopped
- 1/2 Cup ripe cherry tomatoes, quartered
- 1/2 red pepper
- 1 tsp. cumin
- 1/2 tsp. salt
- dash of pepper
- 1 tsp. chili powder
- 1/4 Cup fresh cilantro, chopped
- juice of ½ lime
- Optional-queso fresco and sour cream

1. Wash the quinoa and put it in a pot with 1 Cup water, bring to a rolling boil. Turn the heat down and simmer until the quinoa has absorbed all of the water, about 10-15 minutes.
2. Meanwhile, carve out a little bit of the avocados to make room for the stuffing. Squeeze some of the lime juice in the avocados.
3. Rinse and drain the beans.
4. Chop the onion, tomatoes and pepper and add to a bowl with the beans.
5. In a small bowl, combine all the spices, cumin, salt, pepper and chili powder.
6. Add the bean mixture with the spice mixture and lime juice to combine everything together. Once everything is mixed well, stuff the avocados with the mixture and top with another squeeze of lime and the cilantro leaves. As an option, also add a dollop of sour cream or a sprinkling of queso fresco.

Roasted Apples, Baked Kale, Baked Sweet Potatoes:

Roasted Apples
- 2 large apples of your flavor choice
- cinnamon

1. Preheat the oven to 275°F
2. Wash and dry the apples. To make slicing easier it may be easier to remove the core first. Cut the apples into thin slices.
3. Place aluminum foil on two baking sheets and spread the apples out around the trays, and then sprinkle the apples with cinnamon.
4. Depending on the apples, it will take from 1-2 hours to bake them. Check the apples for pliability but dryness and flip them every twenty to thirty minutes so that they bake evenly.

Baked Kale
- 1 bunch of kale
- 1 Tbsp. of olive oil
- 1/2 tsp. sea salt

1. Preheat the oven to 350°.
2. Wash and dry the kale. Pull the kale off the stems, tearing into pieces.
3. Combine the olive oil and salt in a bowl and toss the kale in the bowl.
4. Spread the kale evenly over a baking sheet and bake for 10-15 minutes, or until the kale is crispy, but not burnt.

Baked Sweet Potato Fries
- 3 sweet potatoes
- 2 Tbsp. Olive oil

- cayenne pepper
- cinnamon
- salt

1. Preheat the oven to 425°F
2. Peel the sweet potatoes and cut them into long strips.
3. Mix the spices and olive oil together and then cover the fries in the oil mixture.
4. Place on a foil covered baking sheet and bake for 25 minutes, checking for tenderness and turning them over half way through.

Roasted and Spiced Garbanzo Beans
- 1 can or 1 Cup cooked garbanzo beans
- 1 1/2 Tbsp. olive oil
- 1/4 tsp. cinnamon powder
- 1/4 tsp. cayenne pepper
- 1/2 tsp. cumin
- 1/4 tsp. salt

1. Heat the oven to 450°F.
2. Rinse, drain and pat dry the garbanzo beans.
3. Combine the oil and spices in a bowl, then add the beans, mix well.
4. Spread the beans evenly on a baking sheet and bake for at least 30-45 minutes until the beans are crispy.

Kale and Roasted Pepper Bruschetta
- 1 whole grain baguette
- 1/3 Cup olive oil
- 1 garlic clove, minced
- 1/4 tsp. salt
- black pepper
- 1 bunch kale
- 1 red pepper
- parmesan cheese
- 6 oz. goat cheese

1. Preheat the oven to 350°F
2. Thinly slice the pepper.
3. Heat a skillet and gently sauté the pepper over medium-low heat, until caramelized
4. Cut the baguette into thin slices and brush each top with a spoonful of olive oil. Place in the oven for about 10 minutes, you'll know they're done when slightly crispy and tops are slightly brown.
5. In the meantime, wash and pat dry the kale. Tear the kale into small pieces and toss with the remaining olive oil, garlic, salt and black pepper.

6. Put the kale mixture into the skillet on low heat and gently cook until just wilted. Combine the pepper and kale mixtures.
7. Spread the top of each piece of bread with goat cheese, top with pepper and kale mixture and shave parmesan on top.

Roasted Beet, Sweet Potato and Parsnip Salad with Citrus Dressing
(This can also be used as a dinner salad if you add a grain and/or protein side)

- 2 beets, halved and sliced thinly
- 1 sweet potato, halved and sliced thinly
- 1 parsnip, sliced thinly
- 1 Tbsp. Olive oil
- 1/2 tsp. salt
- sprinkling of black pepper
- mixed salad greens, such as arugula, endive, oak leaf, etc. how much is up to you, but start with at least 6 cups
- 1 leek, thinly sliced
- 2 avocados

For Dressing-
- 1 orange, juiced
- 2 Tbsp. fresh minced ginger
- 1 tsp. honey
- 1 Tbsp. olive oil
- dijon mustard, optional
- 1 tsp. white wine vinegar
- salt and pepper to taste

1. Preheat the oven to 400°F and place parchment paper on a baking sheet.
2. Toss the cut-up beets, sweet potatoes and parsnips with the olive oil, salt and pepper.
3. Spread the vegetables evenly on the baking sheet and bake for about 30 minutes, flipping them occasionally. They are done when tender but not too brown.
4. While the vegetables are cooking, mix the salad dressing ingredients together.
5. Wash and dry the lettuce. As the end of the cooking time for the vegetables nears, cut up the leek and avocado and arrange on top of the lettuce. Put the cooked vegetables on the salad. Finally, top with the salad dressing or serve it on the side.

Dark Chocolate Avocado Cookies
- 1 avocado, mashed
- 1 Cup dark chocolate chips or chop up 1 bar of semi-sweet chocolate
- 3/4 cup whole wheat flour

- 1/2 tsp. baking soda
- 1/2 cup sugar or 1/3 Cup applesauce
- 1 Tbsp. vanilla extract
- 1 tsp. cider vinegar
- 1 tsp. cinnamon
- 2 Tbsp. unsweetened cocoa powder

1. Preheat oven to 350°F
2. Mix the sugar and the avocado together until smooth. If you have a food processor, this is a good time to use it. However, if you're using applesauce instead of sugar, simply smash the avocado, by itself, until it's smooth.
3. Mix the applesauce, vanilla and cider vinegar together. Now mix the dry ingredients all together in a separate bowl, everything except the flour.
4. Combine the wet and dry ingredients together and mix well before adding in the flour. Mix until the batter is shiny and smooth and there are no lumps. It is important to have the batter ready before adding the chocolate chips.
5. When the batter is ready, mix in the chocolate chips.
6. Prep for baking by putting a sheet of parchment paper on the baking sheet and drop tablespoons of batter on the baking sheet. Gently shape the cookies into the shape you want them in at final baking time as the cookies don't spread very much in the oven.
7. Bake for 10-12 minutes.
8. Let the cookies finish cooking on the baking sheet for a few minutes and then move to a cooling rack.

Chapter 5: Tasty Vegetarian Recipes for Lunch and Dinner

<u>Southwestern Quinoa Salad</u>
- 1 Cup uncooked quinoa
- 2 Cups vegetable broth or water
- 1 fifteen ounce can of low-sodium black beans, rinsed and drained
- 1 Cup grape tomatoes, halved
- 1 green or red pepper
- 1/2 Cup finely chopped red onion
- 1 jalapeno pepper, finely chopped
- 1 avocado
- 1/4 Cup chopped fresh cilantro
- Juice of 1 large lime
- 1 Tbsp. extra virgin olive oil
- 1/2 tsp. cumin
- Salt and pepper if needed

- *If you have it available to you, cactus is a great addition to this meal.

1. Rinse the quinoa and then drain. Put the quinoa in with the vegetable broth and bring it to a boil. Lower the heat and simmer until all the liquid has been absorbed, about 10-15 minutes.
2. Meanwhile rinse and drain the beans. Cut up all the vegetables and combine them in one bowl. Save the avocado for a topping at the end.
3. Combine the cilantro, lime, oil and spices, whisking together.
4. As soon as the quinoa is done and has cooled down, combine it with the beans and vegetables, finishing by tossing with the dressing and topping with avocado.

<u>Lentil Shepherd's Pie</u>
- 2 onions , chopped
- 1 Tbsp. olive oil
- 2 carrots, chopped
- 2 sticks of celery, chopped
- ¾ Cup of frozen or fresh peas
- 2-3 cloves of garlic, minced
- a small bunch of fresh rosemary
- a small bunch of fresh thyme
- 1 bay leaf
- ½ Cup red wine (optional)
- 2 Cups dry green lentils
- 3 Tbsp. tomato puree

- 4 Cups vegetable stock
- 3 - 4 lbs. of sweet potatoes
- salt and pepper
- 6 oz. Cheddar cheese, grated
- ½ Cup whole milk
- 3-4 Tbsp. butter

1. Chop all of the vegetables and either mince the garlic or put it through a garlic press, combining everything in a medium bowl. Heat a large pot over medium low heat with the olive oil and once heated, add the vegetables. In the meantime, pick the rosemary and thyme from their stalks and chop.
2. Cook the vegetables until tender, about 10 minutes. When the vegetables are ready, add the rosemary, thyme, tomato puree, vegetable broth, frozen peas and lentils. Bring to a rolling boil and then gently simmer for 30 minutes or until you're satisfied with the taste. Don't forget to remove the bay leaf when the mixture is done cooking.
3. Preheat the oven to 350°F.
4. In the meantime, make your potato topping. I'm going to be using sweet potatoes in this recipe. Either cook the potatoes in the microwave (prick all around with a fork first) for about 5 minutes, until soft or roast in the oven at 450°F for at least 45 minutes until soft. When the potatoes are done and cool enough to touch, peel them and mix in the salt and pepper, cheese, milk and butter. Stir everything together well.
5. When the lentil mixture is heated through, spread the mixture in the bottom of a 13X9 inch dish or casserole dish. Top with the potato mixture and spread evenly. If you really love cheese, shred a little more over the top. Cook for about 30-45 minutes, until bubbling.

Sweet Potato and Lentil Chili
- 1 Tbsp. extra virgin olive oil
- 1 onion, diced
- 2 bell peppers, chopped
- 3 sweet potatoes, chopped
- 3 cloves garlic, minced
- 2 Cups vegetable broth
- 2 tomatoes, chopped
- 4 oz. can of green chilis
- 2 Cups cooked lentils
- 2 Tbsp. chili powder
- 1 Tbsp. cumin
- 1 Tbsp. paprika
- Tabasco/hot sauce as needed

- Salt and pepper as needed

1. Use a large saucepan to heat the olive oil on medium heat. Start by adding the onion and bell peppers, and cook until softened but still tender.
2. Add the sweet potatoes and garlic and cook, stirring occasionally, until potatoes begin to soften, but don't burn.
3. Stir in the vegetable broth, tomatoes, chilis, lentils and all of the spices, to taste.
4. Bring to a rolling boil, then reduce heat to medium low and simmer until thickened, approximately 30 minutes, adjusting spices as needed.

Black Bean Veggie Burgers
- 1 can of black beans rinsed and drained
- 1/2 green pepper, minced
- 1 Cup spinach, kale, or both, minced
- 1/2 white onion, minced
- 1/2 Cup corn
- 2 cloves garlic, minced
- 1/4 Cup parsley, minced
- 1/3 Cup pumpkin seeds, chopped
- 1 egg
- 1 Tbsp. cumin
- 1/2 Tbsp. chili powder
- 1/4 tsp. cayenne
- 3/4 Cup bread crumbs
- 4-6 whole grain buns with optional cheese and tomato and avocado

1. Preheat the oven to 375°F
2. Rinse and drain the black beans. Mash the beans well.
3. In a separate bowl, mince the green pepper, onion, garlic, parsley, pumpkin seeds and spinach or kale. Add in the corn and beans.
4. Mix the egg and spices together, then add the mix to the bean mixture. Finally, add in the bread crumbs, mixing well.
5. Form 4-6 patties, depending on the size of burger you prefer.
6. Place the patties on a parchment paper lined baking sheet, and bake for about 10-15 minutes, flip to the other side and bake another 10-15 minutes.
7. A great way to compliment the burgers is to toast the buns and add cheese, tomato and avocado.

Quinoa Stuffed Peppers
- 1 Cup onion, chopped

- 2 Tbs. olive oil
- 1 Tbs. ground cumin
- 2 cloves garlic, minced
- 1 Cup spinach or kale
- 1 small zucchini, chopped
- 2 plum tomatoes, chopped
- 1 fifteen oz. can black beans, rinsed and drained
- 1 Cup uncooked quinoa
- 1 Carrots, minced
- 2-3 Cups grated cheese of your choice, low fat, full fat monterrey jack or cheddar divided
- Salt and pepper
- 6 large bell peppers, halved lengthwise, ribs removed

1. Rinse the quinoa and put in a pot with 2 ½ Cups of water.
2. Bring the water to a boil. Lower the heat and simmer until all the water is absorbed, approximately 15 minutes.
3. Preheat oven to 350°F.
4. Heat the oil in a saucepan over medium heat. Add the carrots and cook 5 minutes, or until soft. Then add zucchini and garlic, cooking another 2-3 minutes.
5. Add tomatoes, cumin and spinach or kale and sauté 1 minute until wilted.
6. When the vegetable mixture and quinoa are done, stir everything together, including the black beans and 1 Cup of the cheese. Add salt and pepper if needed.
7. Fill a small amount of the bottom of the baking dish with water.
8. Fill the bell peppers with the quinoa mix and put in the baking pan. Cover the dish with aluminum foil and bake for 1 hour.
9. Uncover the baking dish, and sprinkle the remaining cheese on each pepper. Bake an additional 15 minutes, or until the cheese has browned.

Sweet Potato Mac and Cheese
- Whole wheat pasta of your favorite shape
- 3 Tbsp. unsalted butter
- 3 Tbsp. all-purpose flour
- 2 Cups of milk, whole preferred
- 1 large sweet potato, cut into small cubes and cooked
- 2 Cups shredded cheese, either a blend or cheddar
- Fresh sage, chopped
- Salt and pepper as needed

1. Preheat the oven to 350°F.

2. Peel and cut the sweet potato into small cubes. When the oven is hot enough, put the sweet potato onto a baking sheet and cook for 30-45 minutes, until tender.
3. Meanwhile, bring a pot of water to boil and cook the pasta.
4. In a sauce pan over medium low heat, melt the butter, but don't let it brown. Add the flour and whisk constantly for 2-3 minutes, turning down the heat if necessary.
5. Add the milk in a steady stream, stopping after 1 cup and continuing to whisk for 2-3 minutes. Add the second cup of milk, still whisking and cooking for another few minutes while it thickens. Add the salt and pepper.
6. Add in the cheese and stir until smooth. When the cheese mixture is ready, add the cheese, sweet potatoes, sage and pasta together and gently stir.
7. Depending on how crispy you want the mac n cheese, either put in a 9 by 13 or 8 by 8 inch dish and top with more cheese if desired. Bake for 25-30 minutes.

Black Bean, Sweet Potato and Avocado Enchiladas
Sauce
- 2 Tbsp. extra virgin olive oil
- 2 Tbsp. all-purpose flour
- 1 Tbsp. chili powder
- 2 Cups water
- ½ tsp. cumin
- ½ tsp. garlic powder
- ½ tsp. onion powder
- ¼ tsp. cayenne pepper
- ½ tsp. salt
- 2 tsp. unsweetened cocoa powder

Topping
- 1 ½ Cups of Monterey Jack or cheddar or whatever cheese you like

Filling
- 1 (15 oz.) can black beans, rinsed and drained
- 1 avocado, cubed
- 1 medium sweet potato, cubed into small pieces
- 1 small tomato, chopped
- 4 scallions, sliced
- ½ Cup cilantro, chopped
- ½ tsp salt
- 6 small flour tortillas (whole wheat if you can find them)

1. Preheat the oven to 350°F.

2. Cube the sweet potato into small pieces. When the oven is ready, put the cubes on piece of parchment paper on a baking sheet and bake for 30-45 minutes, until tender.
3. Prepare the sauce by whisking together the olive oil, flour and chili powder over medium heat until it starts to bubble. Whisk for 2 minutes, being careful not to let the sauce burn.
4. Pour the water in slowly while continuing to whisk the sauce. Add the spices including the cocoa powder. Keep whisking until the sauce is smooth and simmering and thickens. At this point, it is ready to use.
5. To prepare the filling of the enchiladas, drain and rinse the black beans, then put them in a large bowl. Cut the avocado into cubes, the scallions in slices, chop the tomato, and chop the cilantro.
6. Add everything to the bowl, including the cooked sweet potato, and mix together. Add salt and whatever other seasonings you like.
7. Spray an 8 by 8 inch casserole dish with the non-stick oil spray of your choice. Fill each tortilla with the vegetable and bean mixture and roll them up tightly. Arrange the rolled tortillas in the casserole dish, with the folded side on the bottom. Once the enchiladas are in the dish, pour the sauce evenly over them. Top with the cheese.
8. Bake for approximately 25 minutes, the sauce should be bubbling on the sides of the dish and the cheese browning.

Chapter 6: Delicious and Healthy Smoothies

Smoothies, particularly green smoothies, are a great way to pack the benefits of many vegetables into a single tasty drink. If a smoothie doesn't taste that good to you, adding some of your favorite fruits will almost always help with this. Feel free to experiment with the recipes and make them your own. I make my smoothies with the **NutriBullet Blender**, it does a great job at a reasonable price.

General Green Smoothie Recipe:
- 1-2 Cups of leafy greens, preferably kale, spinach, collards or chard.
- 2 fruits: For example, 1 banana and 1 apple.
- 1 vegetable such as a cucumber, carrot or celery.
- 1-2 Cups Liquid. Water, Milks, Fruit Juices. The amount will depend on how much you want in your smoothie and how much it takes to blend in the fruits and vegetables. It is generally best to use water in the vast majority of healthy smoothies.

Let your smoothie blend for a number of minutes so that it gets creamy instead of lumpy. Another general tip is to use either frozen fruit or ice cubes in your smoothie, which will give it a thicker consistency and can make it even tastier.

Here are a few smoothies that are targeted for specific needs and wants:

Pre Workout: The goal for this smoothie is to keep you hydrated and energized throughout your workout. A good combination of protein, carbohydrates, and fat can help do this. Your smoothie composition will change depending on how you work out and how much you sweat.

-If you sweat a lot during your workouts, consider adding salt or electrolytes to your smoothie.

-Again, depending on the workout, add either 1 Cup of spinach or 1 scoop of protein powder. I prefer pea protein, but there is also whey, hemp, soy, etc. to choose from.

A side note as to why pea protein is a good choice amongst the world of protein powders. It is vegan and allergen free as it doesn't have nuts, dairy or soy in it. It is also very easy to digest. However, it is important to note that the benefits from peas in their "natural" state are different than peas that have been processed into the protein powder. According to one study performed at the University of Manitoba in Winnipeg, protein powder not only helps your muscles recover from a workout, but delays kidney disease and can help extend the lives of people suffering from kidney disease.

- 1 Cup frozen or fresh fruit such as mangoes or peaches

- Superfood boost such as Maca powder
- 1 Cup water

Again, let your smoothie blend for a number of minutes.

After Workout: The goal for this smoothie is to hydrate and let your muscles recover. A combination of carbohydrates and proteins is needed.
- Scoop of protein powder. Once more, I prefer pea protein, but whey, hemp, soy, etc. are also fine
- Frozen banana
- Spinach
- Almond or Soy milk (an easy to digest milk, so no dairy)
- Other fruit if needed for the taste, or add a natural sweetener like agave, honey, dates or raisins

Muscle Building: For after workout
- Scoop of protein powder
- Ground flaxseed
- 1 Cup low fat/reduced fat Greek yogurt
- 1 frozen banana
- 1 Cup other frozen or fresh fruit if needed
- 1 Cup greens, such as spinach
- Dates
- 1 Cup water

Weight Loss: This is a meal replacement smoothie so it doesn't need to be added to a meal, it should be used solely as a meal:
- Protein powder
- Banana
- 1 Cup frozen or fresh mixed berries
- 1 Tbsp. Chia seeds
- lowfat Greek yogurt
- 1 Cup water or almond milk

Stomach Soother:
- 1-3 Tbsp. Ginger
- 1 Cup frozen or fresh papaya
- Yogurt
- Ice

Immune Booster
- Orange, Strawberries, Cantaloupe or Pineapple
- Banana, Mango
- Kale
- Almond Milk

As you see from all of these recipes smoothies are easy to make and you can alter the ingredients to fit your specific tastes or needs. Feel free to experiment and come up with your own favorite recipes.

Chapter 7: Fitness Tips for Vegetarians

Water
It's always a great idea to drink lots of water. I highly recommend ZeroWater, I have tried all sorts of different water sources and types and think that ZeroWater is the best value. You can also buy the filters in bulk to save a little money. ZeroWater Filters. Drinking lots of water is one of the best things you can do for overall health and fitness.

Peak Performance
If you find that you are lacking in energy, feel that you could be more productive, or just need more discipline and willpower, be sure to check out my bestselling Peak Performance E-Book series: Ultimate Energy, Influence, Willpower, and Discipline, and Ultimate Productivity.

Protein
"But where do you get your protein?" is almost always the first question people ask when talking to a vegetarian. It's actually very easy, especially if you don't have food sensitivities. Let's begin with some of the foods that are excellent sources of protein and readily available throughout the world.

-Tofu and Tempeh
-Nuts (especially walnuts and almonds)
-Seeds (especially hemp, chia and flax)
-Quinoa
-Eggs
-Greek Yogurt
-Lentils and Beans
-Vegetables (especially Spinach and Peas)
-Protein Powder (Whey, Hemp, Pea, etc.)

Considering these options, one can engage in the same workout as anyone else on a different diet. Drinking the protein smoothies I recommend earlier in the book helps restore and build muscle. Weight gain, specific types of training, and other fitness routines call for high protein intake, which these foods can easily provide. So you can build just as much muscle on a vegetarian diet than someone who is eating lots of meat. The below guide can give you a sense of the ratios contents you may want to consider, especially when working out.

40-50% Carbs, 25-35% protein, 20-30% fat
45-65% Carbs, 10-35% protein, 20-35% fat
*Endurance athletes need to eat more calories

I will close this chapter with a few detailed recommendations targeted at specific parts of fitness routines. For more intense workouts, there are recommended pre and post workout snacks for endurance during the workout and recovery afterward. Some of the smoothie recipes mentioned earlier are great for this.

Pre workout-3 parts Carbohydrates to 1 part Protein plus a bit of healthy fat. This ratio will provide an instant boost of carbs as well as longer sustaining release from protein.

Post workout-No dairy because it is hard to digest. Drink something like a protein smoothie within 30 min of working out when muscles are best ready for recovery. The ideal carbohydrates to consume are high-glycemic index carbohydrates like raisins, bananas and dates. You will want to replace glycogen lost and give muscles protein they need. Combining proteins and carbohydrates within the first 30 minutes after exercise is important and beneficial because this combination greatly increases the body's insulin response. Insulin is important because it stops the use of fat as an energy source. Insulin is also needed in the blood to remove too much glucose.

Conclusion

I hope this book was able to help you start off as an informed vegetarian or refine and spark new ideas as a current vegetarian.

The next step is to take what you've learned from this book and turn it into action. You can do this a number of ways including designing your meals ahead of time and making bulk batches of your favorite foods. Start eating a lot more fruits and vegetables and just see how great they make you feel. If you can keep it up for a few weeks you should start to see some noticeable improvements in your life. Once you make it a habit, it becomes much easier to maintain over time and you will be much healthier.

Being a vegetarian is not a diet that has to limit you. There are many easy ways to keep yourself healthy with a whole new world of delicious and healthy meals. As you embark on or continue the adventure of vegetarianism this book can be used as a guide for you return to over and over for your favorite recipes. If this is your debut as a vegetarian, you'll quickly see how easy it is to substitute another protein for meat. It is an experience and lifestyle full of many rewards.

Finally, if you discovered at least one thing that has helped you or that you think would be beneficial to someone else, be sure to take a few seconds to easily post a quick positive review. As an author, your positive feedback is desperately needed. Your highly valuable five star reviews are like a river of golden joy flowing through a sunny forest of mighty trees and beautiful flowers! *To do your good deed in making the world a better place by helping others with your valuable insight, just leave a nice review.*

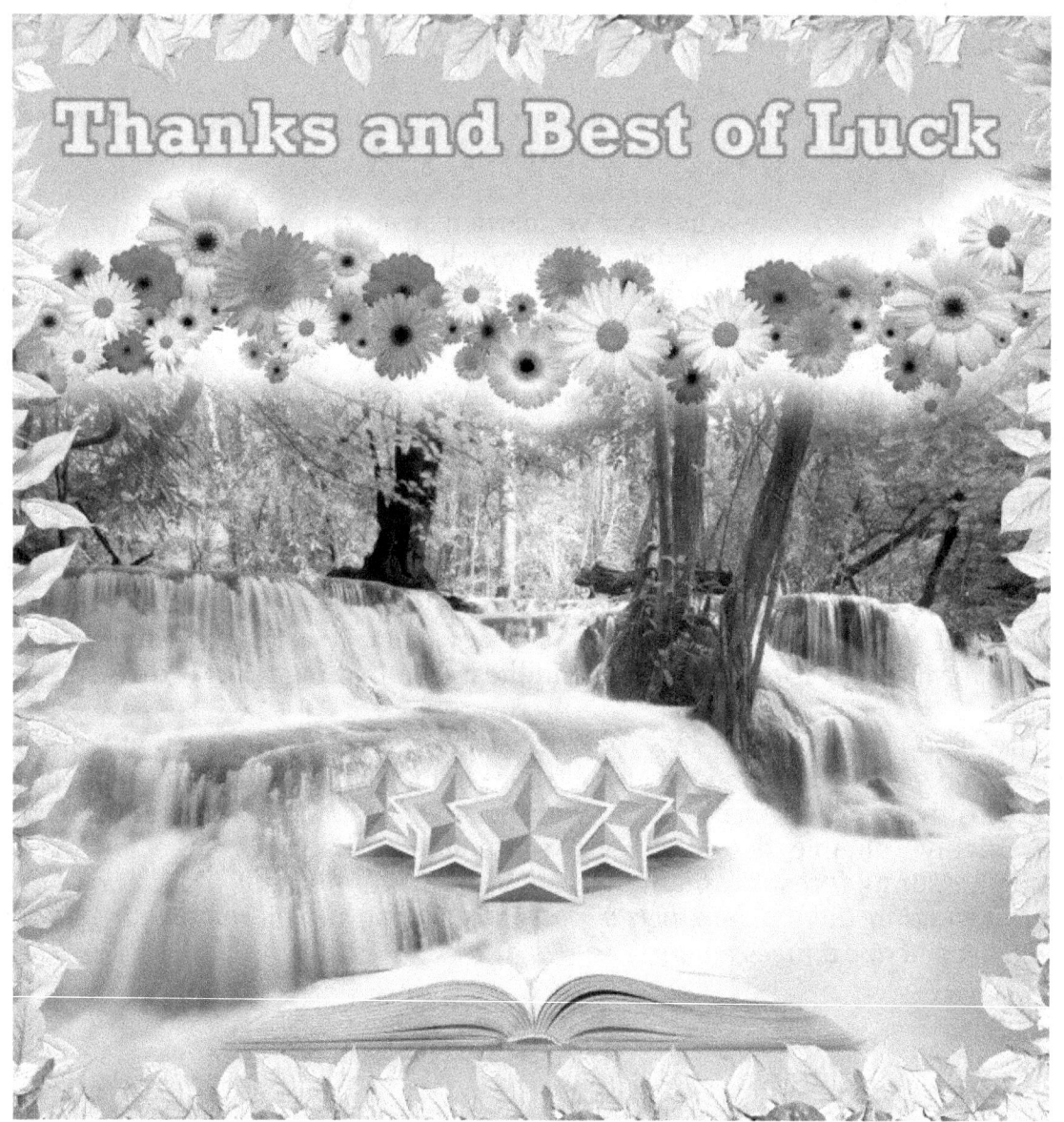

My Other Books and Audio Books
www.AcesEbooks.com

Health Books

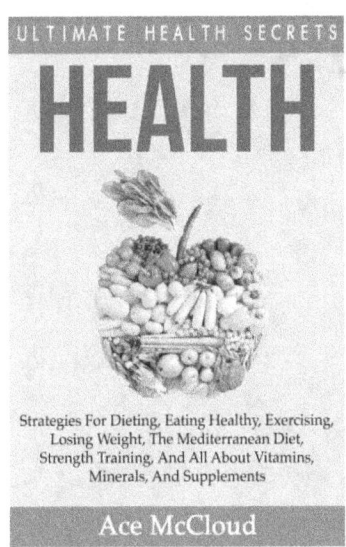
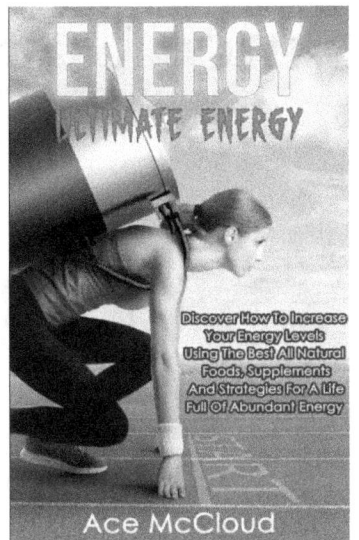
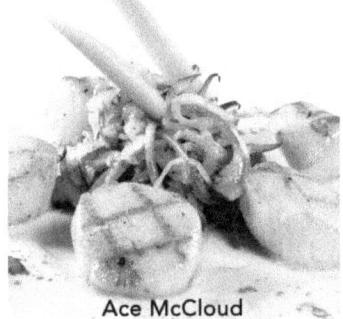
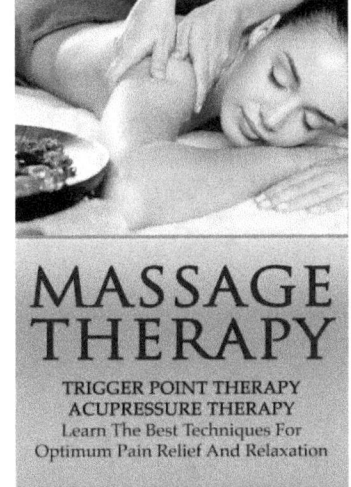
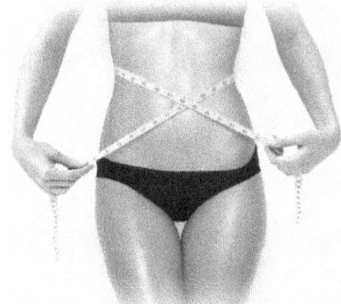
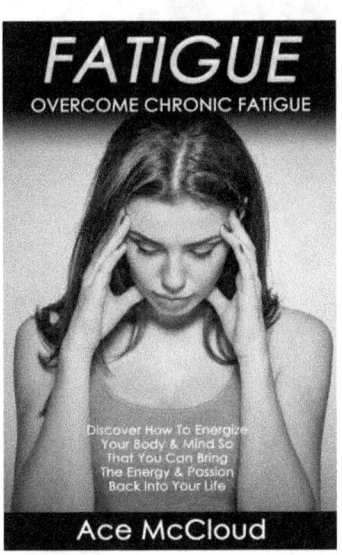

Peak Performance Books

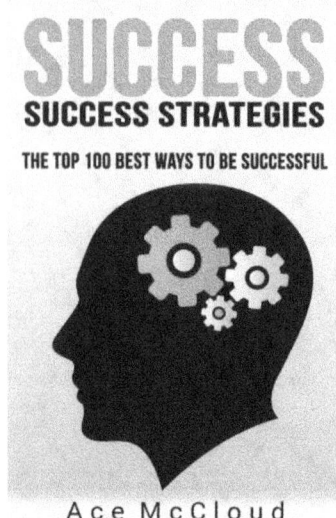
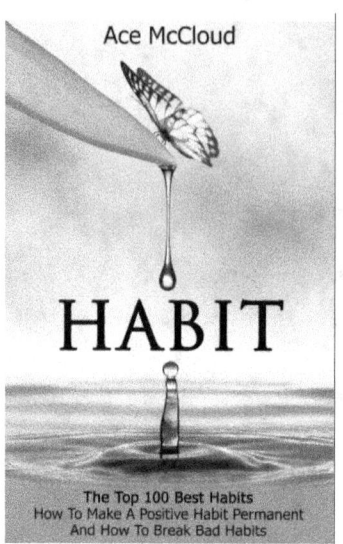
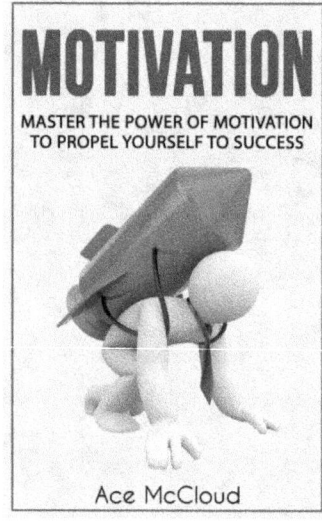
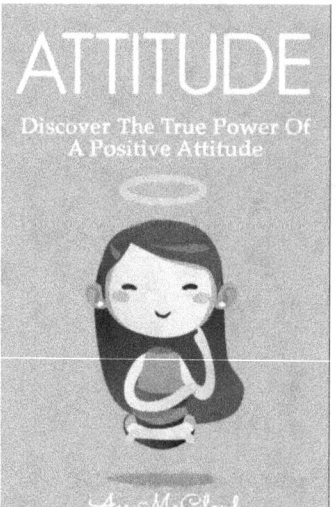

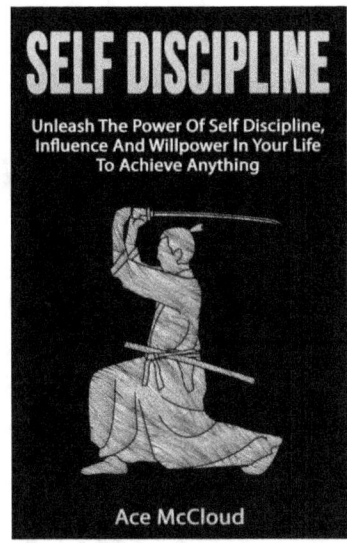 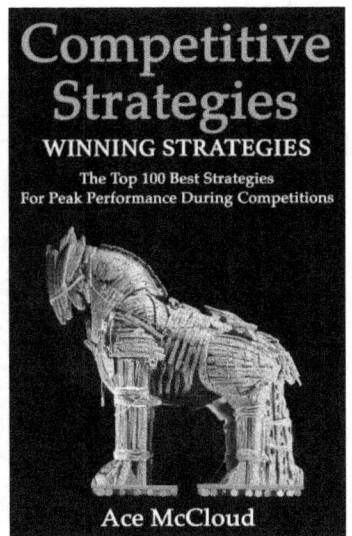

Be sure to check out my audio books as well!

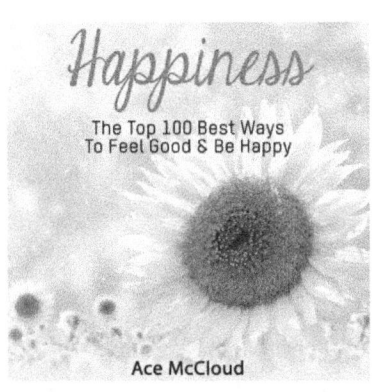 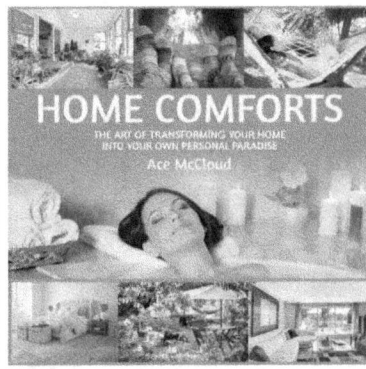 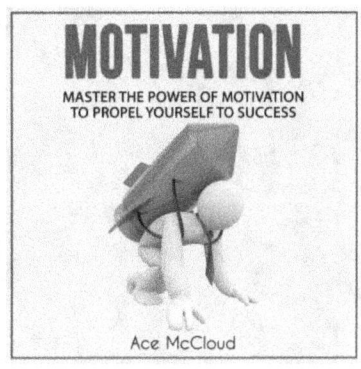

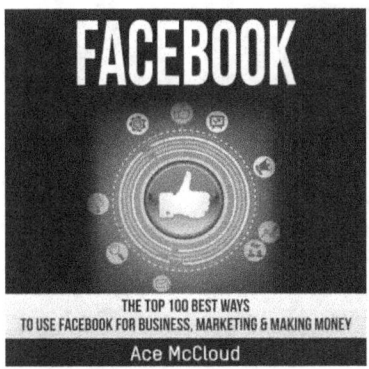 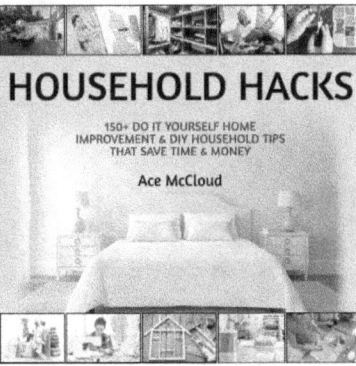 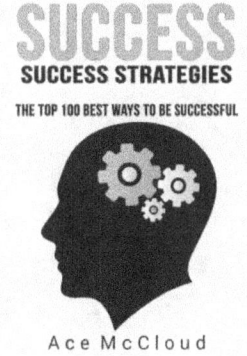

Check out my website at: **www.AcesEbooks.com** for a complete list of all of my books and high quality audio books. I enjoy bringing you the best knowledge in the world and wish you the best in using this information to make your journey through life better and more enjoyable! **Best of luck to you!**

www.ingramcontent.com/pod-product-compliance
Lightning Source LLC
Chambersburg PA
CBHW051428070526
44584CB00023B/3630